Hacks for good health and prosperity

Ways to attain proper health care

Table of content

Chapter 3-Hacking Happiness

Introduction

Life is busy. It might be exhausting to work hard, play hard, and then work even more. Additionally, finding the time for exercise, proper diet, and "brain space" that we require to lead healthy, fulfilling lives can be challenging.

The risks of leading this lifestyle are

numerous and diverse, ranging from fatigue to anxiety to heart disease. It's time we stopped and thought about ourselves.

It's simpler stated than done. To assist you improve your health, we asked our experts for some simple and quick life hacks.

You don't need me to tell you that finding the motivation to always eat healthfully and frequently exercise is difficult. Though we don't always recommend taking the simple road, there are situations when health-related life hacks are useful. You know, little tips and methods that don't take much work yet make remaining healthy and fit simple, and that can improve, balance, and potentially even lengthen your life.

Tittle

1.United health group

2.Carteret health care

3.Texas health care breeze urgent care

4.Life hacks for good health

5.Simple health hacks

6.Ways to wish good health

7.How to keep heart healthy and strong naturally

Chapter 1

Diet hacks

The fact is that dietary adjustments nearly often have an even greater influence on weight loss than exercise.

However, you don't have to give up carbohydrates or go vegan in order to experience benefits.

Here are some

quick tips for improving your diet instead:

Keep a food journal. Studies show that keeping track of your food consumption can help you lose weight and keep it off. However inaccurate it may be, calorie tracking can be effective. It's simple thanks to apps like

MyFitnessPal and Lose It! Additionally, Withings offers a range of gadgets for tracking physical activity, vital signs, and sleep patterns.

Get rid of the trash. Put an end to whatever you're doing and drop everything you don't truly need to.

Rather than canned, choose

fresh or frozen. Cans of vegetables, soups, and beans have increased salt content. Furthermore, canned fruits frequently contain extra sugar, negating the majority of their health benefits. Fruits and vegetables that have been frozen keep more of their nutritious worth.

By doing this, you can obtain your smoothie, scrambled eggs, or snack without having to go shopping right away.

When eating, turn off the TV and get up from your computer. While eating, watching TV (as well as movies or TV shows on your computer) is linked to overeating and making poorer food choices. Additionally, the ads for junk food and beverages don't help. So take a break and, when you can, concentrate on your meal.

Fruit should be utilized in place of sweets. In general, fruit is far superior to typical desserts as a sweetener. Fruits can also include fiber and antioxidants, which will help you avoid the dreaded after-meal sugar slump. It's also fantastic and virtually always a choice when dining out.

Do not rush. Our bodies may not recognize when they are full when we eat quickly, which leads to overeating. The digestion of most foods takes at least 20 minutes. Therefore, take your time while eating, slow down, think before grabbing seconds, and stop when you're satisfied.

Remain hydrated. There are surprisingly many advantages to drinking a lot of water that have been supported by science. By reducing your overall energy consumption and enhancing metabolism, it aids in weight loss.

You can consider this a fitness tactic as well because a fascinating research of soccer players revealed individuals who drank hydrogen-rich water before vigorous exercise also had more energy as a result of lower blood lactate levels.

You should fine yourself for misbehavior. Tell

your friends to gently approach you when you engage in bad behavior, and when you are caught, give them a dollar. Exercise, abstaining from alcohol, and other behaviors you desire to modify will benefit your money.

One of the simplest ways to improve your

health is to eat more fruits and vegetables. Although our consumption has increased, a recent Nutrition and Diet Survey indicated that we still only eat an average of fewer than three pieces per day.

Making a fast smoothie is a terrific way to consume a lot of fruit and veggies all at once. Smoothie makers that also function as travel mugs are becoming more and more common, and if you shop about, you can find one for a really good price.

Also, try not to have the same old things all the time. A good rule of thumb is to go for different coloured fruit and vegetables in your smoothies when you can. Include lots of berries, fruits and superfoods like spinach are another great addition to a smoothie. Also remember dried, canned or frozen fruit or vegetables can be part of your regular smoothies. It's easy to have lots of frozen fruit in the freezer and throw a handful into your smoothie maker each morning.

Chapter 2

Fitness Hacks

Make fitness a regular part of your life; it goes without saying that this is one of the best things you can do for your general health. In fact, studies have shown that even light exercise can boost your energy levels, lessen exhaustion, raise your capacity for creativity, and improve your focus and decision-making. The following tips will help you stay motivated and get the most out of your workouts:

Maintain a regular training schedule. According to research, starting an exercise routine in the morning can help you stick with it. But if you're not a morning person, don't worry about it. If you are consistent, your body will adjust to exercise at any time of day.

Visit the gym during off-peak hours. Avoid going to the gym when it's most crowded because that's when everyone else is utilizing your favorite equipment and weights. Off-peak exercise times result in less waiting, fewer traffic, and a more effective workout. (Bonus points if you go in the middle of the workday to increase productivity!)

Instead, use your own weight as resistance. No gym? No issue. Bodyweight exercises entail working out against your own weight. They are practical because they don't need special tools and can be carried out practically anyplace. They're also great for strengthening the structure of your body, and depending on the activity and the quantity of repetitions, they may be readily customized to meet your unique needs.

One of my favorite, most underappreciated forms of training is bodyweight work.

Find ways to exercise while

traveling. Other typical justifications for skipping a workout include "I'm too busy traveling" and "I can't find a gym on the road." You may find the closest commercial gym with apps like Gymsurfing (currently only available in San Francisco), while GoRecess lists the finest local fitness classes. Not interested in leaving the hotel? You can get fitness coaching from well-known applications like Nike Training Club,

FitStar, and Daily Burn. Without the need for a gym, GAIN Fitness, Power 20, and Sworkit will produce quick and simple bodyweight exercises you can perform wherever you are.

Join a class with others. You dislike working alone? When attempting to begin (and maintain) a new exercise plan, we can all use some help. When you exercise in a group, you get to meet people who are going through the same things as you and can relate to your hardships. Consider enrolling in a class in yoga, spinning, or Japanese samurai sword fighting. Setting up a specific time to work out will help you stay on track, and the class and instructor will act as an integrated support system.

Play some music.

Unbelievably, listening to music can help with performance, motivation, and distraction reduction in addition to being a cure for boredom. The "rhythm response," or how much a music makes you want to move, and tempo of a song are the most crucial elements of a workout playlist. Although music with a beat rate of roughly 160 beats per minute is typically preferred by runners, the motivational effects seem to plateau about 145 beats per minute. Here are the top 10 workout music to get you started (according to Spotify, at least).

At work, move around more and stand. Long hours of sitting increase obesity, bad posture, and chronic discomfort, according to ongoing research. Using a standing desk at work can help you spend less time sitting down. Try to conduct any weekly meetings while walking to reduce stress and blood pressure (among other awesomeness).

Find a workout partner. Having a buddy or

coworker who is participating in the same fitness program can bring accountability, encouragement, and pleasure, just like attending a class. One study found that practicing with someone who is physically fitter than you yields even greater benefits. According to a different study, people can still benefit from having a virtual training partner.

Employ a trainer. Do you find it difficult to exert yourself in the gym? According to research, working out with a trainer can boost your motivation and workout intensity. A client's attitude may also improve as a result of working with a trainer, according to one study. Trainers aren't always inexpensive, but if you're determined to invest, be sure the purchase is worthwhile.

Put your words into action by deeds. If your money was on the line, would you be more motivated to exercise? The Pact app, which encourages you to achieve your eating, eating well, and exercise goals by investing a modest amount of money in yourself, makes that guarantee.

swear a ton of sh*t. Researchers looked at whether swearing increased pain tolerance, which may sound strange. Some of the subjects actually profited from it, mostly as a result of the "fight or flight" impulse it triggered and the resulting physical responses. Don't assume having a potty mouth will make you feel better; instead, channel your rage into constructive goals like setting new personal bests in the gym. Upon further investigation, it was shown that the amount of cursing has a decreasing effect on pain relief. Perhaps a "U.S.-based short sh*t-ton" rather than a "metric sh*t-ton," then.

Try to picture the exercise.

According to research, even just visualizing yourself finishing that last set or half-mile will assist your body be ready to execute it.

Although it seems absurd, it is real.

Run a race. Since you have a specific objective to strive toward and a deadline for completion, signing up for a fun run is a good way to start a fitness program. Visit Active to look through nearby races. One of my favorite races is the Color Run!

Chapter 3

Hacking Happiness

According to research, your emotional state has a significant impact on your health. Stress and other unfavorable emotions might actually weaken your immune system. Consider how your brain might be affecting the rest of your body when trying to enhance your health.

Here are some suggestions for simplifying that:

Put it in writing. Writing down our thoughts and feelings may help us feel less stress throughout the day, according to research. Writing down difficult memories can help them lose some of their power. If they're good, writing them down might increase your sense of gratitude. So grab your Moleskine!

Take a shower before retiring. Before going to

bed, a warm shower helps lower body temperature and inhibit metabolic processes including heart rate, breathing, and digestion.

Due to a decrease in body temperature, it may even aid in sleep. (It's also a fantastic location to allow your thoughts to wander and generate ideas.)

Have some chewing gum or dark chocolate. Your metabolism is stabilized and the stress hormone cortisol is controlled by dark chocolate. Gum chewing also lowers cortisol levels. I feel happier just thinking about these!

Time spent outside (or at least look at pictures of nature). In addition to the numerous physiological benefits of exposure to sunlight, going outside for 15 minutes each day has been related to improved mental health.

Positivity,

happiness, and emotional stability can all be increased simply by gazing at photographs. Meditate. The amount of evidence that demonstrates the health advantages of meditation is astounding, but don't be put off by it as I was. Starting with well-known programs like Headspace and Calm.com is quite easy. There are also a ton of surprising ways to delve deeper when the time is right.

You may be able to manage stress and high blood pressure, get better sleep, feel more balanced and connected, and even reduce your risk of heart disease by engaging in mindfulness and meditation practices.

Meditation and mindfulness are

practices that can help you let go of stress and feel more at ease and peaceful. These practices frequently involve breathing, quiet reflection, or sustained attention on something, such as an image, phrase, or sound. Consider it a brief break from the tension in your life! Your body's natural alarm system is stress. Your breathing quickens, your heart rate increases, and your blood pressure goes up as a result of the hormone adrenaline that is released. It motivates us to act, which is advantageous when we are in a real danger or have a task to do.

www.ingramcontent.com/pod-product-compliance
Lightning Source LLC
LaVergne TN
LVHW080554160826
845677LV00010B/1847
9798355960544